A Womans
GUIDE
TO A HEALTHIER NEW YOU

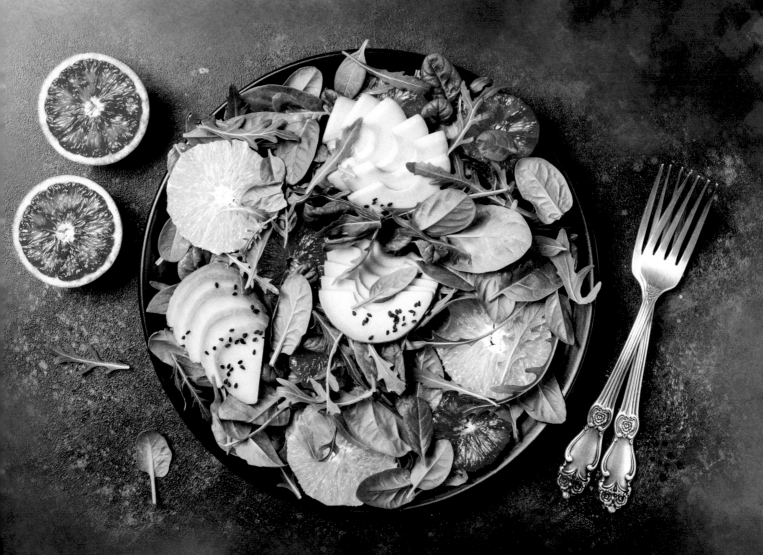

DR. PERDITA FISHER

Welcome

Thank you for supporting this simple guide to a more radiant, vibrant, energetic you.

While on this journey, we will explore your core beliefs about health and wellness, identify traits and habits that keep you on the food and fitness roller coaster ride, excuses that keep you from maintaining the momentum that you want and need to be your best self every day.

During the course of my time in private practice as a dentist, I saw many patients who came to me with a long list of problems and a bag full of medicines. Some of my patients experienced emotional, mental, and other fears about the dental experience and health in general.

As I began to study nutrition due to some health issues of my own, I realized first hand the impact of the mouth/body connections that many speak of today. During the early years, it was not popular to relate disease in the mouth to the rest of the body. Nor was it popular to look at the function of the teeth, including our salivary glands, or our digestive system due to what we put in our bodies. We certainly did not think about what we put on our bodies, or the thoughts or conversations we allowed to enter our minds. As a result of the light bulb in my mind. I decided to include other aspects of wellness into our dental practice. These included acupuncture, massage and esthetical services, hypnotherapy, reflexology, a "30 days to a healthier you detox program", and seminars on wellness in our center. Initially, the main focus was on food. But as I have evolved in my personal development, I realized that there were other barriers that needed to be explored on the journey to wellness.

I have coached men and women on becoming healthier, but I chose to focus on women because of my personal experiences that relate to the feminine connection.

I will share stories and lessons learned. I encourage you to find a friend or buddy with shared goals to help you both stay encouraged and accountable. This is a journey, not a destination. There are no mistakes, just choices we make.

This journey will require sacrifice, discipline and realistic goals that you choose for

YOURSELF!

"OUR POWER IS IN OUR WORDS. OUR POWER COMES FROM TAKING RESPONSIBILITY FOR OUT LIFE." -LOUISE HAY

WHAT'S INSIDE

So, do you want to become a Healthier version of you?

If being healthy us your goal, you must align your behavior with that objective. Your habits and environment must be connected with health, healing and wellness. Health involves mental, physical, social and spiritual elements. Haven's we all heard the express "you make me sick?"

We can really become sick by constantly being in the company of negative, complaining people. Thoughts of envy, malice, lies, deception, jealousy… are just some vibrations that adversely affect out cells. A merry (happy) heart is better than medicine.

We have been mis-educated about health. Is the health of our community getting better or worse? New diseases that we can't pronounce are increasing. We have a legacy of parents that outlive their children. We have more doctors, hospitals and legal drug dealers (like Walgreens and CVS) on every corner.

We have taken Physical Education out of many schools, and video games and fast food restaurants are the new norm. We bought into this new sedentary lifestyle. Our ability to think has been compromised.

Whatever steps you Decide to make toward change, applaud yourself. The longest journey begins with the first step. Take the first step to take charge of your own destiny. Surround yourself with positive people and get onboard.

As a woman thinketh, so is she. Our inner world reflects out outer world. Our thoughts have so much power. But to change our outer world, we must start within. The process of change begins in the mind with intention.

Today, more than ever, we must be mindful of what we consume, physically, emotionally, and psychologically. The things that we consume can either enhance and improve our health or can cause an unhealthy degenerative cycle on our health. There is an abundance of negative information that can and will affect our immune system.

"OUR POWER IS IN OUR WORDS. OUR POWER COMES FROM TAKING RESPONSIBILITY FOR OUT LIFE." -LOUISE HAY

Mindset Is Key

Mindset is key to Awareness. Let's look at our Beliefs and Mindset.

Debbie Ford says "all suffering is from saying one thing and doing another".

This is incongruent behavior. For example, I said I would work out at noon but I got a Facebook notification that kept me engaged for hours and I did not work out.

We must cultivate a mindset to keep moving even with ups and downs. If we don't show up for ourselves and transform our thoughts, who will?

How do we get to that transformation? Let's look at Limiting Beliefs:

Limiting beliefs may come from many areas in many forms such as parents, teachers, media, etc. Examine what you inherited from others that is not true, for example you are slow, or fat. The Lizard Brain is the center of our lack of progress. It protects you from what you want but don't know how to get.

When the lizard brain shows up, we make choices that lead us on a path away from our big goals. The Lizard Brain shows up as:

- Procrastination
- Distractions
- Excuses

Now that we have identified how the lizard brain operates, let's identify your origins of limiting beliefs so that you can install new empowering beliefs.

Your Assignment:

Write your success story as if it already happened. What did you learn from your Mother about health and wellness that no longer is true for you?

- Your Father?
- Your Grandparents?
- Your Teachers, Friends, or Media?
- Write it down.

For each limiting belief, write an empowering belief to replace it.

- Keep it in front of you, read it or say aloud until you really begin to really embrace the new thought habits.
- Focus on what you want instead of what you don't want
- Shift your language from I have to... to I choose to…
- Act as if success is certain. Do whatever it takes.
- Live your life based on your values and not others.

Personal Note: I have written affirmations for most of my life. But the words did nothing to transform me because I did not own them. I did feel the emotion for the words I spoke. Even when I looked in the mirror, I did not see me as the words I was reciting. So, remember our words must equal the feeling, otherwise the brain does not believe us. Change did not occur until I attached the emotion (feelings)to my words.

"OUR POWER IS IN OUR WORDS. OUR POWER COMES FROM TAKING RESPONSIBILITY FOR OUT LIFE." -LOUISE HAY

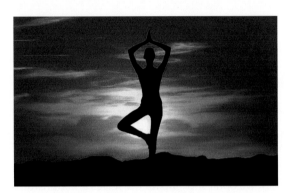

Breathing & Meditation

Now that we have created new beliefs about wellness, let's look at Breathing and Meditation. When we were born, breathing was natural and rhythmic. As we aged, our breathing became shallower and more labored due to stress and racing thoughts.

Breathing is the simplest form of meditation and can easily be done any time. Breathing is a key component to health. The goal of breathing is to allow the mind to rest from thoughts. Does anyone suffer from racing thoughts? If you are like me, the answer is yes. I had to practice breathing techniques for months to re-learn what once was intuitive.

Here are 3 breathing Techniques: Try each one to see what works best for you.

1. **The 4-7-8 Breath**
   Place the tip of your tongue against the ridge of tissue just behind your upper front teeth and keep it there during the entire exercise. You will be exhaling through your mouth around your tongue; Exhale completely through your mouth, making. a whoosh sound. Close your mouth and inhale quietly through your nose to a mental count of four. Hold your breath for a count of seven. Exhale completely through your mouth, making a whoosh sound to a count of eight. This is one breath. Now inhale again and repeat the cycle three more times for a total of four breaths. If holding your breath is difficult, you may speed it up, making sure to keep the ratio of 4:7:8.

2. **Soft Belly Breathing**
   Let gravity pull your shoulders down. Place the palm of your hand on your relaxed belly. Slowly and deeply inhale, allow your abdomen to expand, and notice the hand on your abdomen moving outward. As you exhale, move your belly button back toward your spine and notice your hand moving inward. Repeat three times, and pay attention to any shifts in your body and your level of relaxation.

3. **Left Nostril Breathing**
   Sit comfortably. Close your right nostril with your right thumb, stretching your other fingers straight up. Close your eyes and begin to breathe long and deep, only through your left nostril. Continue for three minutes.

Personal Note : My breathing was always shallow and I didn't realize my patterns until I saw and began to practice these techniques. When I feel tense or nervous, breathing brings me back to a state of calm. I do a rapid fire breath in the morning to energize me and I love the 4-7-8 breath at bedtime. It helps me focus on my breath and let go of the day. For me, twice a day and the stress goes away!

Meditation

There is no right or wrong way to meditate. In the beginning, you may find it difficult to slow your mind and tap into your inner consciousness. You might want to begin in the morning before beginning your daily tasks.

Meditation comes in many forms such as prayer, chanting, breathing, ritual exercise, viewing art or listening to music. The goal of meditation is to allow your mind to be still. Meditation works best when practiced daily. Begin with short meditation so that you stay consistent. Even if you begin with 5 min a day at the same time every day.

As you experience the benefits, experiment with new types. Meditation will help slow your mind, allowing you to tune into your intuition and live in deeper alignment with your intentions.

Meditation Tips:

- If possible, avoid eating one hour before meditating
- Sit in a comfortable position
- Close your eyes and sit quietly for a few seconds.
- Introduce a mantra (a specific thought) if desired.
- Take a deep breath and express gratitude at the end of your meditation.

There are many resources for meditation. I have used Deepak Chopra, Mediations via podcast, or other audio meditations.

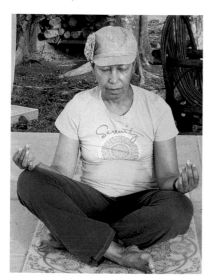

Other resources for Meditation:
- Headspace app – approx. $13/month for 20 min meditation
- Deepak Chopra- www.chopra.com
- www.mindspace.org
- www.mayoclinic.org/meditation
- Dr Weil's Breathing Basics- http://geti.in/1bjcAY77
- Parul Epstein's Happiness through Meditation- http://geti.in/WJT7pr
- Muse Headband- approx. $200

Personal Note: Meditation was very challenging for me at first. It took a long time to quiet my mind. My mind was always racing. I learned to focus on my breathing when a thought interrupted my focus. The mantra really helped to deepen my experience. I include some form of meditation in my life at least twice a day.

Elimination

Toxins are everywhere; In the environment, in foods, in conversations and in some of the people that are in our lives. Accumulations of toxins can affect our mood, energy and general well-being. Common causes such as constipation, poor diet, overeating, lack of water, stress, antibiotics, late night eating and lack of exercise are all contributors.

Toxicology textbooks list the first symptoms of chronic poisoning as low energy, fatigue, muscle weakness, inability to concentrate and intestinal complaints. These symptoms are the same as those experienced by the chronically ill. Unfortunately, in our polluted environment, many bodies become overloaded. This could result from exposure to environmental toxins even before birth. It can be the result of lifestyle habits such as poor diet, drugs and alcohol or the result of toxins in the body itself.

Regardless of the cause, the bottom line is that for most people, the body's systems can't process the toxins as quickly as they are ingested or generated. Factors such as stress or unresolved emotional issues, or other illness can impact the immune system which is our body's defense against illness in individuals.

The good news is that you can improve and protect your health by implementing your personal detox program. Detox is a state of mind. You will not succeed unless you make up your mind to do so. You will need self-discipline to resist unintentional temptations from friends, families, co-workers, or advertising. Consumable toxins will tempt you to " eat me", personal care toxins will say "these smells so good but contain harmful, artificial ingredients not designed for the skin or body. The visual and the aromas draw us in.

For women, as the detox process intensifies, emotional and physical issues may get worse before you feel better. The self-awareness and understanding are mental processes that accompany the physical process. But rest assured that the detox process will help bring you back to a physical state that will improve your body, emotions and ability to concentrate and make self-sustainable decisions.

Let's set some SMART (Specific, measurable, attainable, realistic, time sensitive) Goals: Identify the goals you have set for a higher state of well-being:

Do you want to eliminate processed foods, reduce sugar consumption, drink more water, add a new fitness routine, associate with people that share your values, or let go of people and things that no longer serve you?

Whatever the goals are, write them down, be specific, review them weekly and adjust if needed. I will plan my menu and grocery list every Sunday at 1 pm for the following week.

Personal Note: I usually will make a menu plan for the week . I shop early in the day and prep for 3 days at a time.

Preparing my lunch for the next day after dinner keeps me from rushing before going to work and eliminates the urge to eat processed foods or foods that are not healthy simply because I failed to plan. I also make a practice to remove myself from toxic conversations and energy. Other people's negativity affects me physically and mentally. I realized I can not change anyone's thoughts or perceptions so I had to set limitations so I could eliminate the drain it placed on me.

A few elimination techniques such as dry skin brushing and castor oil packs are detailed on the page to follow.

Dry Skin Brushing

The Skin is the largest organ of the body.

The benefits of dry brushing your skin include:
- Moving lymph
- Increasing energy
- Supporting the body's ability to detox
- Improving cellulite

The Technique

Begin with your feet, brushing upward with long strokes toward the heart. Brush each area 5-10 times to get the maximum effect for the lymphatic system and detoxification.

Move to your legs, thighs, stomach, armpits and back, brushing in a clockwise motion on each section, toward the heart one section at a time.

Your face should be the last place you brush. Switch to a softer brush if available.

Your skin should be a light pink without pain or irritation. If you have pain or irritation, use less pressure or a softer brush.

If you want to get your blood flowing, you can use dry brushing every morning before your hot lemon water or before showering. I like to do at night also before a soaking Epsom salt bath with lavender or other essential oils

Castor Oil Packs

The benefits of Castor oil packs include:
- Happy hormones
- Supports digestion
- Improve circulation
- Supports healthy skin
- Helps the detox process
- How to make a castor oil pack

This can be messy, so make sure you use an old towel or blanket to lie on.

Materials:
- Several layers of flannel to cover the stomach or other affected area
- A high-quality bottle of castor oil (from the health food store)
- Plastic wrap larger than the flannel by about two inches on all sides
- Hot Water Bottle (or heating pad)
- Container with a lid that can hold the flannel (I use a large jar with wide lip or storage container or gallon size bag)
- An old towel or blanket

Steps :
1. Place the flannel into the container and saturate it with castor oil. It should be covered and moist all over without dripping excess oil back into the container.
2. Prepare the area where you are going to lay by setting out an old towel or a blanket; If castor oil drips beneath you, it will stain so protect your couch, bed or chair. (I usually lay on the floor on a blanket and towel)

Food & Mood

Food has a big impact on our mental and emotional well-being. For many people, food is also associated with certain memories and emotions. Complete the following to explore how food and mood are related in your life.

- When you think of your childhood, what role did food play in your family?
- Write about any memories you have related to eating/food and love or nurturing.
- Write about any negative associations you have with food, ie. bad memories.
- When/if you use food to manage your emotions, what specific foods do you use:
- For sadness?
- For anger?
- For fear?
- For stress/anxiety?
- When you are tired?

Personal Note: If chips, cookies, or processed foods are in my physical space, it's tempting so to avoid the temptation of eating mindlessly, I leave them in the store. I once tried hiding them from myself, but it didn't work. Out of sight, out of mind. Don't you feel lighter now that you have installed new empowering beliefs?

Essential Tips For A Successful Cleanse

Remind yourself of why you are doing this and the benefits you will experience. Have everything you need: Stock your fridge with foods you can enjoy and get rid of the foods you need to avoid?

Eat Mindfully: Sit with no distractions and enjoy every bite of your food. Chew slowly and properly as digestion begins in the mouth.

Increase Fiber Intake: Whole Grains, fresh fruits and vegetables especially leafy green vegetables. Eat foods high in beta carotene, Vitamin C and Vitamin E. Include a variety of each.

Drink plenty of water: 70% of your body is water. Water also serves as a transporter for energy. Drink at least half your body weight then continue to add up to 120 ounces daily. Proper hydration will help flush out toxins from the body, and keep you feeling full.

Move your body: Exercise is important to any cleansing regime. Moving your body stimulates your lungs, blood and lymph circulations and your liver and lymph nodes. Your digestion is stimulated, you sweat out of your skin, your kidneys filter the contaminants. Movement can be as simple as a brisk walk.

Limit Electronics: This includes phone, computer and TV exposure.

Relax: Take this time to relax by enjoying a bath with essentials, Epsom salt or clay. The warm bath will help you prepare for a good night's sleep. It might be helpful to keep a food diary to help you evaluate your habits around food. Simple recipes will be added in this guide but I encourage you to order the "Breath of Life Detox "book by Vanessa Williams, for the Breath of Life Detox Program.

It includes the what, when, how and why including a daily guide.
https://checkout.square.site/buy/Q3H7K2WSXG2SENI255PUJ7IE

You can contact me for a 3 day or 30 day program.

Personal Note: I like fasting at least 8 hours one day a week from solid foods as a part of the cleansing process. I also practice Sugarless week and Live Foods week 4 times a year with the change of each season. I find that cleansing with the change of seasons is in harmony with nature and is life enhancing.

Assimilation

Take time to do what makes your soul happy.

Practice Relentless Self Care

S- Self talk positivity

E- Exhale and Inhale

L- Look for the healthiest food available and look for something positive daily

F- Find joy and gratitude in everyday experiences

C- Connect with nature everyday possible and connect with community

A- Appointment with yourself

R- Rest, Restore, Relax, Renew and Replenish

E- Experience Every Day as an opportunity for a New Beginning.

Evaluate Every Area of Your Life for Balance

1. **Spiritual** : Meditate, sing, dance, pray, practice self-forgiveness, self-reflection, find spiritual mentor or spiritual community
2. **Personal**: Learn who you are, decide what you want in life, make short and long-term goals, create a vision board, Relax, spend time with loved ones, Learn something new.
3. **Emotional**: Practice self-love and compassion, Laugh, Affirmations, Say" I Love Me and Hug yourself, schedule quiet time on your calendar. Set limits
4. **Psychological** : Journal, self-reflection, acknowledge your positive qualities, ask and receive help, Read or listen to self-help books, join a support group
5. **Physical** : Eat healthy real foods, Exercise, get adequate sleep, take vacations, Create "me" time regularly.
6. **Professional:** Set boundaries, leave work at work, take regular breaks, Say No, take a class, get support from colleagues, leave the building.

Personal note: I grew up thinking that it was selfish to love yourself on a daily basis. Self-care was reserved for "special" occasions like birthdays or anniversaries, and included massages, nails, etc, modeled by my mother and grandmother. Now, I know it's not selfish, it's necessary. If we don't put our mask on FIRST, we can't help anyone else. I often worked so much that I made myself physically sick. I am grateful that I learned that Self Care is necessary before it's too late. Now, I schedule a date with myself on my calendar. I get excited to be with ME. I hope that you will too.

Treat Your Body Like A Sacred Temple Affirmations

- My body deserves the best; I consider the impact of everything I put into my body
- I enjoy exercising and I know my body is healthier when I make exercise a part of my life
- I make healthy choices and I avoid activities that risk my health

Habit Trackers:

1. Sleep- Get deeper, more restorative sleep
   a. eliminate caffeine after 2 pm
   b. Get outside early for melatonin production and sleep in dark room
   c. Remove visible stressors such as papers, laundry
   d. No screens before bed and keep regular bedtime.

"Sleep is the golden chain that binds health and our bodies together" Thomas Dekker

2. **Move**
   a. Calf Stretch
   b. Power walk
   c. High intensity cardio 2 hr before bed aids mood and sleep
   d. Break every 60-90 minutes

"Exercise should be regarded as a tribute to the heart"- Gene Tunney

3. **Increase Energy Levels**
   a. Smile and Laugh often
   b. Plan and set goals
   c. Drink more water
   d. Eat protein

Be Kind to yourself, you are doing the best you can

4. **Improve your digestive health**
   a. Eat fermented foods
   b. Consume fiber
   c. Reduce snacking and low nutrient processed "instant" foods
   d. Intermittent fasting

Our Food Should Be Our Medicine and Our Medicine Should be Our Food "- Hippocrates

5. Fuel your Fitness Goals
   a. Eat when hungry, stop when full
   b. Add vitamin d3 supplements and get out in sunshine
   c. Eat a light snack after workout
   d. Drink water

Eating Well is a form of self-respect

6. Learn something New Every Day!
   a. Listen to podcast or audio books
   b. Ask & Answer questions
   c. Remember- memory games and exercises
   d. Expand your outlook and desires

"Exercise of the Muscles keeps the body in health, and Exercise of the brain brings peace of mind". – John Lubbock

7. Nurture a Healthy Mindset!
    a. Keep a gratitude journal
    b. Meditate
    c. Reflect on your success
    d. Expand Personal development

"Gratitude makes sense of the past, brings peace for today, and creates a vision for tomorrow" - Melody Beattie

8. Morning Practices for balance
    a. Wake gently and practice breathing fully
    b. Move your body
    c. Meditate
    d. Prioritize

"A healthy outside begins with the inside"- Robert Urich

9. Monthly Restorative Habits
    a. Celebrate wins
    b. Add new foods
    c. Disconnect EMF exposure & negativity
    d. Create new goals

"Each choice starts a behavior that over time, becomes a habit"- Darren Hardy

10. Create your own Habit

Tips For A Clearer, Focused Mind

1. **Change your breakfast. Instead of cereals and bagels, try a smoothie.**

    To make your shake habits easier:
    - Use a time of day that is best for you to prepare (use can arrange ingredients to blend and drink
    - the next morning.
    - Rotate all vegetables, fruit, liquid and spices at regular intervals
    - Use a powerful blender like the Vitamix or Ninja for maximum creaminess

2. **Stop Multitasking;** Allow yourself to focus on one thing at a time .
3. **Consider the medications you are taking.** Are changes in medications affecting your memory?
4. **Increase healthy fats in your diet. (**Add 1 tbsp of coconut oil daily or avocado)
5. **Eliminate processed sugar from your diet.**
6. **(Pay attention to your symptoms; they could be sending you a message)**

Affirmations

- I resist junk food.
- I enjoy eating healthy. I cook for my family and myself. Preparing food at home gives me more control over what we put in our bodies. I cut down on sugar, salt, and unhealthy fats. I find recipes that taste delicious and fit the time I have available.
- I carry my own snacks. I like my treats better than the candy bars and chips in my office vending machines.
- I pause before indulging. I ask myself if a donut is really worth the calories. The impulse often passes if I wait a few minutes.
- I avoid emotional eating. I manage stress by taking a walk or talking things over with a friend. I celebrate special occasions without stuffing myself.
- I think critically about advertising. I make my own decisions instead of ordering pizza because I see a commercial on TV.
- I sleep well. Junk food is less tempting when I feel well rested.
- I shop wisely. I avoid going to the grocery store on an empty stomach. I spend most of my time browsing the outer aisles so I can pick up vegetables and yogurt without looking at candy and frozen dinners.
- I eat before I get too hungry. I have more willpower when I feel full.
- Today, I fill up on delicious whole foods instead of empty calories. A healthy diet gives me energy and helps me to lead a long and happy life.

Self-Reflection Questions

1. **How can I reward myself with things other than food?**

2. **What are some environmental triggers that make me crave junk food?**

3. **How does eating junk food affect my health?**

Personal note: Years ago, I bragged about being able to multitask as a great accomplishment. I was so wrong! Typing while talking on the phone often found me typing what I was talking about. I later experienced burnout from trying to juggle too many things at once. I am still learning that efficiency and proficiency is better than speed. I started doing the easier tasks first so I could have a feeling of accomplishment. Now I have shifted to begin with the most important things first early when my mind is fresh. A fresh smoothie made with sunwarrior collagen energizes me and helps me focus.

You can find sunwarrior products at perditafisher.com/servicesandresources for 15% off..

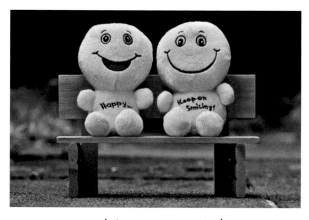

Tips For A Better Life

1. 1. Walk 10-30 minutes daily. Smile while you walk.
2. 2. Sit in silence at least 10 minutes each day.
3. 3. Drink plenty of water.
4. 4. Make at least 3 people with a smile each day.
5. 5. Eat more foods that grow on trees and plants and less food manufactured in plants.
6. 6. Avoid negative thoughts, energy vampires, issues of the past and anything you can't control.
7. 7. Invest your energy in the positive present moment.
8. 8. Complete the following statement when you wake, "My purpose is to _____ today.
9. 9. Life is what you make it, make it good.
10. 10. Life is too short to waste time on hateful negative energy.
11. 11. Don't take yourself so seriously
12. 12. Agree to Disagree. You don't have to win every argument.
13. 13. Make peace with your past so it won't spoil the present.
14. 14. Don't compare your life to others. You have no idea what their journey is about.
15. 15. Take charge of your own happiness.
16. 16. Look at every "so-called" disaster with these words: In 5 years, will this matter?
17. 17. Forgive self, Forgive others.
18. 18. What other people think is none of your business.
19. 19. Stay in touch with your friends.
20. 20. Envy is a waste of time. Use your time wisely.
21. 21. You are too blessed to be stressed
22. 22. Guard your time- leave room for unscheduled hours
23. 23. Use your power within to create your own reality.
24. 24. Learn something new every month.
25. 25. Complete the following before going to bed: I am thankful for _____.
26. 26. Today I accomplished_____

Additional resources:
- Plantrician Project
- Forks Over Knives
- Veg Fund
- Abillionveg

Books:
- Ageless Vegan
- By Any Greens Necessary
- Breath of Life Detox
- The New Soul Vegetarian Cookbook

Videos:
- What the health
- The Game Changers
- Cowspiracy
- Fat, Sick & Nearly Dea

Personal Note: I have been practicing affirmations for many years.. Initially, I could not look in the mirror . I have found that mirror work is essential. I needed to see myself and feel the emotions of me being who I know I am . Sometimes through tears, I spoke positivity to me until I could learn to smile at myself in the mirror as I loudly proclaimed my value and worth. You can too.. Look for something to be grateful for every day.

Peaceful Getaways:
www.ghanedenbz.com

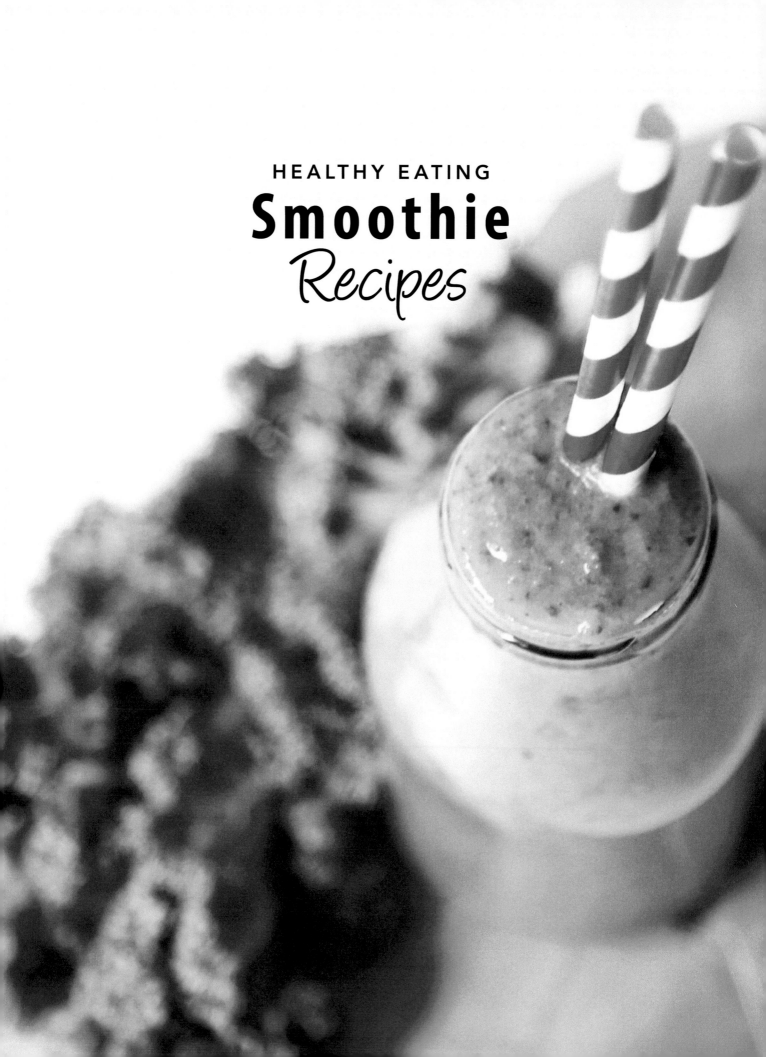

HEALTHY EATING

Smoothie
Recipes

01 Smoothies

INGREDIENTS

- ½ c frozen organic cherries or other berries

- 8 oz of fermented coconut water, coconut water or filtered water

- 3 Tablespoons of collagen as a protein base (Sunwarrior has a great plant-based collagen protein powder.

- 1 Tablespoon of sprouted nut butter or sun better1 tablespoon coconut oil

- 1-2 tablespoons of raw cacao or cocoa powder

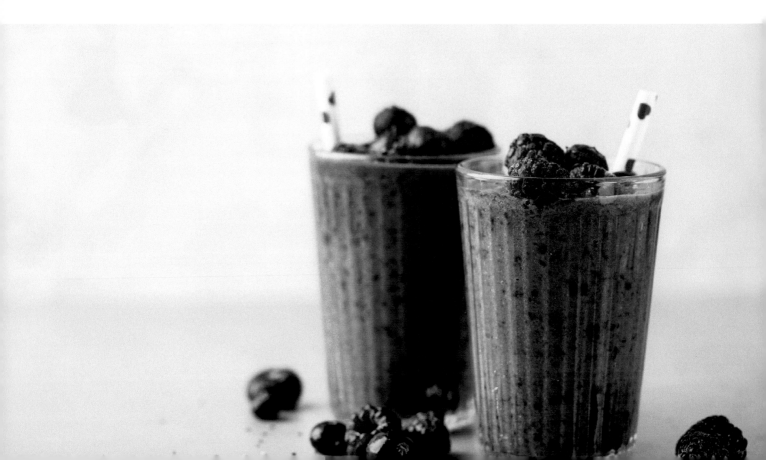

02 Anti-Inflammatory Blackberry (Blueberry) Sunrise

INGREDIENTS

- Handful of spinach

- 1 cup frozen organic blackberries or blueberries

- 1 can or box full fat coconut milk

- 3 tbsp raw cacao powder

- 1 scoop protein

- 1 tbsp turmeric

- Pinch pink salt and pinch cayenne pepper

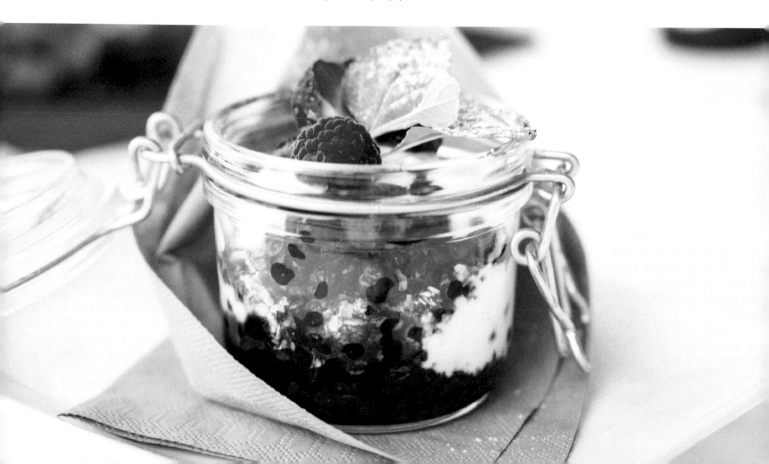

03 Coconut Crunch Super Shake

INGREDIENTS

- 1 cup coconut milk
- 2 tbsp almond butter
- 2 scoops protein powder
- ¼ cup raw cacao nibs or dark chocolate chips
- 1 tsp vanilla stevia if desired

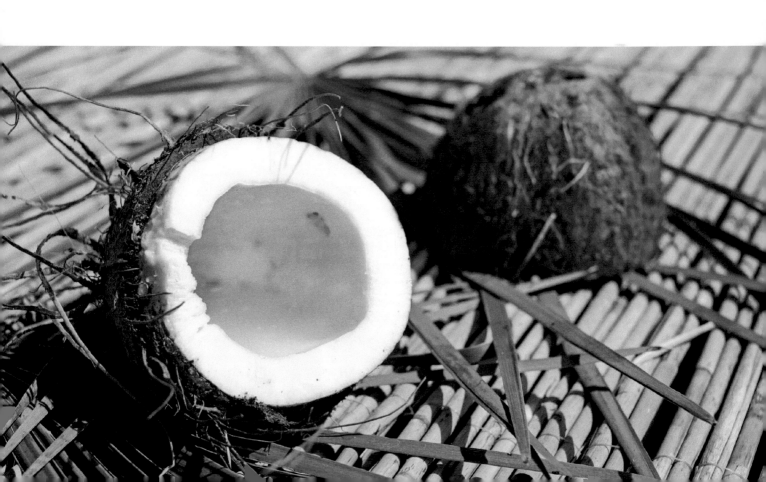

04 Chocolate Chia Super Brain Shake

INGREDIENTS

- 1-2 cups organic almond or coconut milk (carton)
- 1 tbsp raw cacao powder
- 1tsp chia seed
- A scoop of high-quality protein powder
- ½ avocado
- Ice-optional

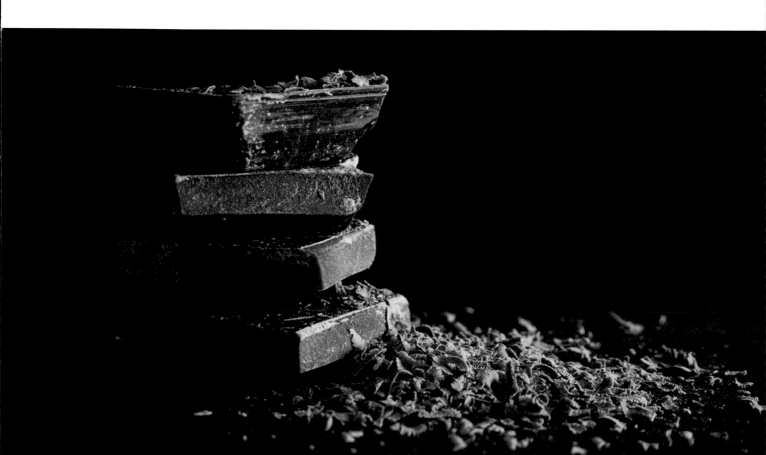

A Prayer From Me To You

My Prayer is that you love yourself no matter what, no matter how, now matters when. If you get off track, take a deep breath and start again. You might have bumps and bruises, mis-steps and failure but use these as tools for learning and stepping stones to your next level. The life you really want to live is on the other side of fear and doubt.

You have within you the power to create your own reality. Claim the life and health you deserve today!

Enjoy this adventure to a healthier new you.

- We choose to be healthy
- We choose Joy
- We choose Happiness
- ALWAYS Choose YOU!

When the mind, body and emotions learn to nourish themselves by embracing the wisdom of the spirit, Love prevails. Enjoy the journey called life.

Love,

Dr. Perdita Fisher

PS. REMEMBER:
- Begin with a Decision- Take Action
- Master Yourself- spend time with you; be gentle with yourself and you go deep inside'
- Move out of your comfort zone- FREEDOM is beyond your fear!
- Trust the universe and the process; the process is a lesson
- Enjoy the journey- Never arrive; there is always the next level up called Ascension
- Be coachable, teachable and practice
- See yourself as if you are already there.
- Breathe, pray, Meditate, Journal, Affirm, Visualize and BE the Best YOU!

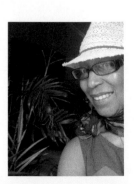

FOR MORE INFORMATION

PERDITAFISHER.COM

To order additional copies of this book, contact:
Xlibris
1-888-795-4274
www.Xlibris.com
Orders@Xlibris.com

ISBN: Softcover   978-1-6641-2364-9
        EBook   978-1-6641-2363-2

Print information available on the last page

Rev. date: 08/18/2020

For more information about my projects, products, and services please visit the following :

https://linktr.ee/HEALTHIERNEWYOU
https://perditafisher.com
https://www.ghanedenbz.com
https://www.amazon.com/author/perditafisher

Printed in the United States
By Bookmasters